Entomological field techniques for malaria control

PART II

Tutor's Guide

World Health Organization
Geneva
1992

WHO Library Cataloguing in Publication Data

Entomological field techniques for malaria control.
      Contents. pt. I. Learner's guide — pt. 2. Tutor's guide

      1.Anopheles   2.Entomology — education   3.Malaria — prevention and control   4.Mosquito control —
      methods   5.Teaching materials

      ISBN 92 4 154439 2 (pt. I)   (NLM Classification: QX 18)
      ISBN 92 4 154440 6 (pt. II)

© World Health Organization 1992

TYPESET IN INDIA
PRINTED IN ENGLAND
91/8904—Macmillan/Clays—5500

Contents

Preface

This training module on entomological field techniques for malaria control is in two separately bound parts. The first part is the Learner's Guide, containing technical information; Part II is the Tutor's Guide, which provides advice for those responsible for conducting training programmes.

The module is one of several[1] being produced by the World Health Organization, each concerned with a different aspect of the control of malaria. It can stand alone as a medium for the training of public health workers engaged in entomological field work for malaria control or it can be used as part of a longer and more comprehensive training programme on malaria. The need for such a module was identified by the Member States of the World Health Organization, and it was developed by Mr J.L. Clarke in collaboration with the Programming and Training Unit of WHO's Malaria Action Programme. The original illustrations were meticulously prepared by Mr Yap Loy Fong of Kuala Lumpur, Malaysia. The text has been revised on the basis of observations and suggestions made by many people, in particular by Dr McWilson Warren, former Team Leader of WHO's Interregional Secretariat for the Coordination of Malaria Training in Kuala Lumpur, Malaysia, and by staff attached to that unit, notably Mr P. Blizard, Professor C.Y. Chow, Dr Han Il Ree, Professor B. Richter, Mr J. Storey and Dr Suwan Wongsarojana. The text was finally modified by Dr. P.F. Beales, Dr C.W. Hays and Dr. D. Muir.

WHO expresses appreciation to all who have assisted in the preparation of the module, and wishes to acknowledge the collaboration and financial support provided by the United States Agency for International Development in this and other activities of the Interregional Secretariat for the Coordination of Malaria Training.

---

[1] Already published: *Basic malaria microscopy* (1991).

Introduction

This Tutor's Guide is designed as an aid to those responsible for running training programmes in entomological field techniques for malaria control. As such, it has two purposes:

- To assist in the planning, organization, and implementation of training activities.
- To assist you, the tutor, to teach as effectively as possible. To this end, it offers a set of guidelines that you can follow in helping learners to become as proficient as possible in the various field techniques. These guidelines can be adapted to suit the facilities you have available, the requirements of the entomological services in your country, the learners' needs, and your experience and skill as a tutor.

Training based on this module is designed to teach the learners a number of entomological collecting techniques, and to help them to understand the importance of correctly performing the tasks involved. Examples of such tasks are the distinguishing of female anopheline mosquitos from other species and the collecting of female anopheline mosquitos inside a house. Each task has been analysed in terms of the knowledge, skill and level of competence that learners must acquire, and each is the subject of a general learning objective set out in this Guide. More detailed learning objectives are given in the Learner's Guide (Part I of the training module) and are not repeated here. However, you are strongly advised to read and become familiar with the Learner's Guide before planning and implementing a particular training activity. At the beginning of each teaching session, you should remind the learners of its objectives.

Organizing the training programme

The details given in this section are based on a number of assumptions and are intended to represent an ideal situation. If the resources and facilities available to you differ from those described, you will need to modify and adapt your training programme appropriately.

The training programme should last for between three and four weeks. It is designed to teach individuals with no previous experience or training in malaria work.

The number of participants in the training programme should be limited to 20. They should all have had at least six years' formal schooling, although previous experience of mosquito collecting work may be acceptable in place of a certain amount of school education. Participants should all be in good general health and have good eyesight.

As tutor, you will be responsible for the overall direction and coordination of training; ideally, therefore, you will be an entomologist with extensive experience of malaria field work. To assist you, you should have four facilitators, who should be either entomological technicians or health inspectors and who should also have considerable field experience.

The training facility should provide a classroom large enough to accommodate you, the facilitators, and all the learners, plus an entomological laboratory equipped with at least one binocular microscope. For the purposes of lecture sessions and demonstrations, you will require a chalkboard, a 35-mm slide projector, a screen (or plain white wall), an overhead projector, and one or more flipcharts. Additionally, there should be a reference collection of mosquitos, consisting of preserved specimens of adult anopheline and culicine mosquitos, larvae and pupae, and including all vector species that occur in your country or area. Transport for up to 25 people will also be required.

Details of other equipment needed for laboratory and field work are given in later sections of this Guide.

The training facility should be located within a convenient distance of a suitable rural practice area, preferably no more than one hour's drive away. This area should be suitable for the use of all collecting devices (traps, artificial shelters, etc.) and should provide an experimental hut if necessary.

Accommodation facilities for you, the facilitators, and the learners should be available, and suitable financial arrangements should be made for learners to be lodged in field practice areas when necessary.

Principles of the training programme

The training programme described in this Tutor's Guide is based on the following principles:

- Training takes place in the classroom, in the laboratory, and in the field, but the greatest emphasis throughout should be on work performed under actual field conditions.
- Classroom and laboratory work should be confined to the acquisition of essential knowledge and the development of basic skills in collecting and identifying mosquitos, eggs, larvae, and pupae. This should be followed by application of knowledge gained and skills mastered in extensive sessions of field work.
- Effective and efficient learning is encouraged if learners understand the purposes of training and feel that the goals are important to them, to their teachers, and to the community. This is one of the reasons for including the learning objectives in the Learner's Guide.
- Effective and efficient learning is encouraged if learners are actively involved in learning by themselves and from others, as well as from what the tutor tells them. The number of lectures should therefore be kept to a minimum, with learners being urged to find things out for themselves.
- Effective and efficient learning is encouraged if learners can see that they are making progress. It is thus important that the tutor try to understand any difficulties learners may be having and help to overcome them. Regular feedback about their progress should be provided to learners.

Organization of the Tutor's Guide

Each section of the Guide is based on one general learning objective. The sections correspond to the Learning Units of the Learner's Guide and are set out in the sequence in which they might be taught. Specific learning objectives are detailed in the Learner's Guide and are not repeated here. It is important that you elaborate and clarify the technical content of the Learner's Guide by using examples, giving demonstrations and responding to questions. You should therefore be adequately prepared to do this.

- **Equipment and teaching aids**

  A list of minimum essential equipment is suggested to help you in your teaching activities.

- **Teaching and learning methods**

  There are many different teaching methods that you can use and that serve different purposes (see Annex 1). Examples are suggested on the basis of the learning objectives, the desirability of making the training programme as interesting as possible for all concerned, and the need to help learners to learn for themselves.

- **Assessment**

  Both you and the learners should be able to make regular assessments of progress in their knowledge and skills. You are given guidelines on types of assessment that might be used. The methods are directly related to the learning objectives given in the Learner's Guide.

The learning objectives, content, teaching methods, and assessment procedures outlined in the Tutor's Guide may well need to be adapted to suit local circumstances.

General learning objectives for the field collecting of mosquitos

This Guide provides you with many examples of the ways in which you might teach and assess progress in entomological field collecting techniques. It is essential that learners achieve **all** the learning objectives outlined below:

- Understand the tasks involved in collecting mosquitos in the field.
- Understand the basic nature of malaria as a disease and the principles of its control.
- Recognize anopheline mosquitos both as adults and in egg, larval and pupal stages in the laboratory.
- Collect adult mosquitos using a sucking tube (aspirator) and a test-tube in the laboratory.
- Collect indoor-resting adult mosquitos under field conditions using a sucking tube and transport them to the laboratory.
- Collect indoor-resting mosquitos by means of pyrethrin spraying and spray sheets.
- Collect adult mosquitos resting outdoors in natural and artificial shelters, using a sucking tube.
- Collect biting mosquitos at night by direct capture from human and animal baits and prepare specimens for transportation to the laboratory.

- Collect mosquitos at night by means of trap nets baited with human and animal baits.
- Collect mosquitos leaving houses or animal shelters by the use of exit traps.
- Collect larvae and pupae from breeding sites and transport them to the laboratory.

In order to achieve many of these objectives, accurate labelling and record-keeping are necessary for all specimens collected. The particular requirements for these activities are detailed in the relevant sections of the Learner's Guide.

If one of the learners can already perform one (or more) of the essential tasks, his or her training can be modified to take this into account. The more skilled individuals can assist fellow learners to perform particular tasks. Once all the learners have achieved the objectives of a Learning Unit, you can move on to the next Unit of the Learner's Guide.

The following points should be noted with regard to the above list of learning objectives.

- The list is comprehensive, covering all the tasks involved in collecting mosquitos. If, for a particular group of workers, a job description exists that demands training in mosquito collecting, it should be examined carefully so that training can be adapted to provide the necessary skills and competence.
- The sequence in which the objectives are presented has been carefully considered: theoretical and laboratory-based training comes before field collecting, and indoor field collecting precedes outdoor collecting.
- The list of learning objectives may be used to develop a complete timetable for training.

Basic tasks of collecting mosquitos in the field

General learning objective

To acquire an understanding of the basic tasks involved in the collection of mosquitos in the field

In some countries, there is an official job description for health workers responsible for collecting mosquitos in the field. Where this is available, it can be used as the basis for this Learning Unit. If none is available, you should review the basic tasks involved in collecting mosquitos in the field as described in the Learner's Guide. This Unit can be treated quite briefly in a training programme but should not be omitted.

Equipment and support

No equipment as such is required but, if an official job description exists, you will need sufficient copies for each learner to be supplied with one. Otherwise, supply the learners with a list of the tasks involved in field collection of mosquitos.

Teaching and learning methods

Ask the learners to read the job description or the list of tasks you have prepared, then invite queries and comments. You might use this occasion to elaborate on some of the essential elements of mosquito collecting. This brief section will enable learners to see the relevance of the training programme as a whole and to understand its purposes. Returning to this subject from time to time during training will help learners maintain their sense of perspective and ensure that they are all working towards the same goals.

Assessment

No assessment is needed of work done in this Learning Unit.

Notes

Malaria and its control

General learning objective

To understand the nature of malaria and the means of controlling the disease

In this Learning Unit, learners will become familiar with various aspects of malaria as a disease, its transmission by mosquitos, and the methods of treating and controlling it. This will help them to:

- understand the purpose of their work
- answer questions posed by villagers and other people they meet in the course of their work
- understand the importance of taking personal precautions against contracting malaria.

With regard to the entomological collecting techniques described in the Learner's Guide, it should be emphasized that the sampling methods do not attempt to determine absolute numbers of mosquitos but only to estimate their relative population densities. It is for this reason that it is essential to employ standardized methods of sampling.

Teaching and learning methods

Ask the learners to read the text of this Unit carefully, and to discuss it among themselves. You should then ask whether there are any matters they find difficult to understand. Depending on their response, you may choose to give a presentation, lasting not longer than about half an hour, focusing largely on areas where the learners are having difficulty in understanding the written materials.

Guidelines for assessment

Methods for assessing and evaluating learners' progress should be kept as simple as possible. A suitable approach is to use oral or short written questions such as the following:

- Which types of mosquito carry human malaria?
- How is malaria transmitted to humans by mosquitos?
- What are the four stages in the mosquito's life cycle?
- When and where do most anopheline mosquitos feed?
- What are the four kinds of malaria parasite and which is the most dangerous to humans?

- What is drug resistance?
- Why are infants and young children more likely to become sick and die from malaria than adults?
- What is the treatment schedule for *Plasmodium falciparum* malaria in your country?

Role of entomological work in malaria control

General learning objective

To understand the role of entomological work and surveys in malaria control

Equipment and support

Copies of all locally used entomological survey forms should be supplied to each learner.

Teaching and learning methods

Learners should read Learning Unit 3 of the Learner's Guide in advance. You may then ask a range of questions about the purposes of different survey methods used in entomological activities; if the answers are correct, any further work in this area can probably be avoided. The major thrust of your teaching activity should be to underline the necessity of maintaining accurate records of survey data. You may choose to go through each survey form with the learners, explaining the importance of each item that is included.

Guidelines for assessment

Two procedures are suggested for assessing learners' understanding of this Unit:

- Ask the learners to provide written statements of the major purposes of preliminary surveys, operational surveys, spot checks and foci investigations.
- Ask the learners to fill in sets of survey forms for a particular country or region on the basis of actual or hypothetical survey data that you provide. The forms should then be checked for accuracy and completeness.

Notes

Recognition of anopheline mosquitos

> ## General learning objective
>
> To be able to recognize anopheline mosquitos as adults, eggs, larvae and pupae

It is important that learners know how to distinguish between anopheline and culicine mosquitos at all stages of the life cycle because only anophelines carry human malaria. Moreover, since only certain species of anopheline mosquito transmit human malaria, the distinctions between the different species are also important. It is not necessary to know how to identify the species for the purpose of collecting mosquitos, although people doing this work may eventually learn to recognize the main species in the field.

Equipment and support

It is essential to have a well-maintained and adequate teaching collection that contains specimens of all stages in the life cycles of anopheline and culicine mosquitos.

Most of your teaching work in this Unit will require the use of hand lenses, and you should have adequate numbers of these available for the learners. One or two binocular microscopes would be useful, but you should probably limit their use to demonstrations since the present training is not intended to prepare the learners for microscopy work.

It is extremely important that arrangements be made in advance to collect the live material required for laboratory practice in Units 4 and 5.

Teaching and learning methods

In order to help learners to distinguish mosquitos from other insects and to distinguish adult anopheline mosquitos from culicines, it is most important that you first use the drawings given in the Learner's Guide. After the learners have become proficient in distinguishing between the species in the diagrams, they should proceed to study the differences between actual specimens of adult mosquitos, eggs, larvae and pupae. It is comparatively easy for learners to identify the differences using line diagrams, and they can then apply this experience to their work with living or dead specimens.

When you discuss Fig. 2 of the Learner's Guide, it may be useful if you also describe some of the locally prevalent diseases transmitted by other insects: the learners are quite likely to ask about the role of insects other than mosquitos in disease transmission.

In preparing your teaching material and presentations, try to keep the same sequence of information as is followed in the Learner's Guide.

Guidelines for assessment

The following two guidelines will help you to assess whether learners have achieved the learning objectives of Unit 4:

- Present each learner with specimens of at least:
  — five mosquitos and five other insects
  — five male and five female mosquitos
  — five culicine and five anopheline female mosquitos.

  (Recent night catches may provide the samples you need.) Ask all the learners to sort the specimens according to the learning objectives.

- It is important that learners achieve 100% accuracy in this procedure. If a learner makes errors, ask what led him or her to a particular decision. Use the line drawings, or specimens and a hand lens, and point out the distinguishing morphological characteristics. Then test the learner again until total accuracy is achieved.

Similar procedures can be used to assess achievement of the other learning objectives of this Unit: distinguishing the eggs, larvae and pupae of mosquitos from those of other insects, and the eggs, larvae and pupae of anophelines from those of culicines. If learners make errors of identification they should be asked to study Learning Unit 4 again. You should then obtain additional specimens, so that the learners can have more practice in making the necessary distinctions. Conduct further assessments until complete accuracy is achieved.

Hand collection methods and transport of adult mosquitos

General learning objective

To be able to collect adult mosquitos using a sucking tube and a test-tube and to transport live specimens from field to laboratory

---

Equipment and support

No special equipment is needed beyond that listed in the Learner's Guide. However, it is important to stress the need to avoid contamination of material with insecticides when working in treated areas, particularly where residual insecticides have been applied indoors. Indeed, the danger of insecticide contamination should be pointed out frequently during the course.

Teaching and learning methods

Demonstrate how a sucking tube is assembled and how paper cups are prepared. Divide the learners into pairs and get them to demonstrate both procedures to each other. Observe their techniques and correct any errors.

The methods of mosquito collecting are detailed in the Learner's Guide. It is important at this early stage, before the first field trip, to ensure that the learners understand what is required of them and that they are given several demonstrations of the various methods of mosquito collection and transfer. They must then be given adequate opportunity to practise these methods under close supervision: sufficient caged mosquitos must be available for this purpose.

Supervision should focus initially on the collecting methods. When learners have perfected these skills, attention should shift to the transfer of mosquitos; it is important that transfer is accomplished without losing, damaging or killing the mosquitos. Learners can practise both individually and in pairs. When they work in pairs, one learner should observe and comment on what the other is doing; the roles should then be reversed.

If learners can become fully proficient at handling specimens in the laboratory, their later field training will be made easier, quicker and more effective.

It is important to emphasize again the need to label all collections completely and accurately. This is stressed throughout the Learner's Guide but should be constantly reiterated. Encourage the learners to consider the entomological consequences of inaccurate or incomplete labelling; reinforcing the message in this way should ensure that they will always take sufficient care about this aspect of their work.

The maintenance of live mosquitos in the field and during subsequent transportation should be carefully demonstrated. You must emphasize strongly that *live* material is required in the laboratory and that, if many mosquitos are damaged or die during transportation, the time spent collecting them is wasted.

You can help learners to understand the importance of transporting and maintaining mosquitos alive if you:

- carefully demonstrate appropriate methods of packing and transportation, as described in the Learner's Guide;
- supervise the learners in the packing of materials for transportation, and get them to observe and comment on each other's performance;
- ask a laboratory worker to show the learners examples of poorly packed mosquitos and to describe why such specimens are of no use.

Demonstrate how to assemble a killing tube and make sure that the learners can do this. You should emphasize that accurate identification of mosquitos is important and that specimens required for taxonomic studies are collected with killing tubes so that their scales remain intact. Dead mosquitos rapidly dry up and become brittle; they must be pinned quickly while still soft, so that they can be easily examined for external morphological characteristics.

Guidelines for assessment

In the course of your teaching sessions you will already have assessed the learners' ability to assemble sucking tubes and prepare paper cups, so these skills need no further assessment. All assessments should focus on the other basic skills: collecting and transferring mosquitos without damaging them; labelling collections accurately and completely; and keeping mosquitos alive in the field and during transport to the laboratory. During the training pro- gramme all learners should have plenty of opportunities to practise these skills and should become increasingly confident of their abilities. The following guidelines are suggested for the accurate and comprehensive assessment of their proficiency in collecting, transferring and labelling specimens and trans- porting them to the laboratory in excellent condition.

- Ask each learner to collect three samples of five mosquitos using a sucking tube and to transfer them to paper cups without losing, damaging or killing any of them. Learners may practise individually or in pairs initially, but when they come to you for assessment they should collect at least one sample perfectly. A similar approach may be used to assess collection of mosquitos by means of a test-tube.
- Ask the learners to label the collections of mosquitos they have just made. Again, they should be encouraged to work individually and to obtain feedback from each other and from you. When they choose to present themselves for assessment, however, complete accuracy is required.
- Ask each learner to collect a sample of mosquitos and to keep them in a paper cup overnight. Examine the specimens the next morning. If there is a high mortality rate, try to determine why and provide feedback so that the

learners will be able to pack and transport mosquitos more carefully in the future.

- During the initial field visit, get each learner to pack a consignment of mosquitos for transportation to the laboratory. When the insects arrive at the laboratory they should be inspected as soon as possible. A learner may be judged to have achieved the objective when the combined damage and mortality rates amount to less than 10% of the total sample. (This type of assessment should be made *whenever* the learners send mosquitos to the laboratory, so that the importance of correct packing and transportation is continually re-emphasized.)

Notes

Hand collection of indoor-resting mosquitos

General learning objective

To be able to collect indoor-resting mosquitos in the field by means of a sucking tube and transport them to the laboratory

---

Entomological field work includes the collection of live material either for processing in the laboratory or for use in specific tests, e.g. insecticide susceptibility tests or bioassays.

This Unit covers the learners' first field practice following their introduction under laboratory conditions to the different methods of hand collecting adult mosquitos.

Correct handling procedures for field collecting and for transportation of specimens to the laboratory must be emphasized. Practice is required to ensure that the insects reach the laboratory alive, undamaged and in excellent condition.

Hand collecting is not suitable for obtaining all the mosquitos in a room or structure and cannot therefore be used to determine absolute numbers of insects. However, it does allow the demonstration of seasonal trends in mosquito population densities.

Teaching and learning methods

This will be the learners' first experience in the field and will give them their first contact with the local community. It is most important that you explain some elementary principles of communicating with the people. Most mosquito collecting is done in and around houses, and for this reason the health workers involved must have people's cooperation and permission to enter homes. Explain to the learners that their first step should generally be to contact the community leader or village head. It is essential that they learn:

- whom to approach and how
- how to explain the nature of the work to be carried out
- how to enlist the cooperation and assistance of the community
- how to seek permission to enter private premises
- how to behave while collecting, especially in people's houses.

As organizer of the training, you should contact the local community and secure their permission for your visits before the learners go into the field.

Politeness and sensitivity are essential when approaching people in the community. It is also important that health workers explain to them that mosquito collecting in houses does not cause inconvenience or disturbance. You should emphasize to the learners that they should always be on their best behaviour in order to win people's confidence and cooperation. They should not ask for personal favours, for example the fetching of water. They should not solicit food but may accept it if it is offered spontaneously.

Role-playing is very useful at this stage. Before the learners go into the field, ask one of them to play the role of a villager whose house is to be used for collecting, and another to play that of the health worker collecting mosquitos. These two should act out their parts in front of the rest of the group. The whole group should then discuss the role-play in terms of the principles of effective communication. The procedure serves to build the self-confidence that will be necessary for talking with villagers and winning their cooperation.

Take the learners to the field and let them observe your approach to a community leader. Then visit a few homes, talk to the householders and make arrangements for day- and night-time collecting of mosquitos.

Your demonstrations should consistently emphasize the things that should and should not be done, as described in the Learner's Guide. When learners have returned from the field, give them plenty of opportunities to discuss difficulties they may have had in communicating with villagers. Answer patiently and fully any questions they may put to you.

Each learner should be given the opportunity to practise indoor collecting in at least five houses.

Guidelines for assessment

Assessment should focus on the learners' skill in:

- establishing and maintaining communication and relationships with house-holders
- collecting mosquitos
- labelling and recording collections accurately
- packing and careful transportation of specimens.

The following guidelines for assessment are suggested:

- Observe systematically how learners behave in their communications and relationships with householders. Praise them publicly when they perform well; point out examples of poor communication tactfully and privately, and explain how they could have been improved. Above all, be consistent in demonstrating effective communication yourself, because learners benefit much more from what you do than from what you say should be done. If villagers do not cooperate with workers who are collecting mosquitos, try to assess the reasons for this. Ask the learners to discuss the problem: it may not always be the fault of the health workers. Communication skills are best assessed through observation. Corrective feedback from you and from villagers is important, and learners should be encouraged to help one another to improve their communication skills and develop relationships.

- The learners' skills in collecting, recording and transporting mosquitos in the field can be assessed by similar methods to those used to assess these activities in the laboratory.

Notes

Spray sheet collection of mosquitos

General learning objective

To be able to collect indoor-resting mosquitos by means of pyrethrin space spraying and spray sheets

---

Teaching and learning methods

This Learning Unit is concerned with the acquisition of two new skills: preparing a room for space spraying, and spraying it systematically. The learning objectives also call for the refinement of some skills that have already been acquired in collecting, labelling and transporting of catches.

After obtaining permission from a chosen householder to enter a home, demonstrate the following procedures to the learners:

* clearing small items of furniture
* blocking large openings in walls and ceilings with cloth or netting
* spreading sheets on floors, under tables and beds, and on furniture
* closing windows and doors
* spraying by one person indoors in a well-sealed room
* spraying by one person indoors and one outdoors where cracks and openings cannot be sealed
* the various methods of collecting mosquitos from the sheets.

Note: The pyrethrin spray may have slight residual effects, and the same house should not be used for demonstrations more often than once a week.

While you demonstrate how to prepare a room for spraying and carry out the spraying operation, give a running commentary on what you are doing, and why you are doing it. In particular, emphasize the need for a systematic approach to spraying, as described in the Learner's Guide. Ask one learner to prepare another room and carry out spraying, ask the others to make notes on what is done correctly and what incorrectly. Divide the learners into groups of four or five and ask them to practise these skills. You should pass between the groups and provide them with feedback on their performance.

Opportunities should be given for every learner to develop these skills so that each is able to perform the tasks as an individual rather than as part of a team.

Collecting, labelling and transportation of catches may be dealt with by the teaching and learning methods described in previous Units.

Guidelines for assessment

In this Unit, assessment should focus on the two new skills: the preparation of rooms for spraying and the performance of spraying operations. There should also be further evaluation of the other skills involved, even though these have been assessed previously. The following guidelines are suggested:

- Draw up a simple performance appraisal form as an assessment instrument and give feedback to learners on their skills in preparing and spraying a house and in related activities. An example of such a form is given after these guidelines. It can be used to focus attention on the need for a systematic approach to spraying operations.
- The collecting, labelling and transportation of specimens may be assessed using approaches suggested in earlier sections.

Performance appraisal form for space spraying and spray sheet collection

You should carefully observe what the learner does and complete the form reproduced below. Your observations should be discussed with the learner and used as a basis for improving his or her performance.

	Yes	No	Remarks

Introduction

Did the learner:

- Introduce himself or herself by name to the householder?
- Explain clearly what he/she wanted to do and why?
- Give the householder an opportunity to ask questions?
  Answer them?
- Obtain the householder's permission to spray the house?

Room preparation

Did the learner:

- Select an appropriate room to spray?
- Remove all animals, birds and small items of furniture?
- Remove or cover all items of food?
- Cover all openings and eaves with cloth or netting?
- Close all windows and doors?
- Spread sheets correctly?

Spraying the room

Did the learner:

- Move round the room systematically, in a clockwise direction, directing the spray towards the ceiling?
- Arrange for a second person to spray outside in circumstances where the eaves/openings could not all be covered?
- Spray the room for a suitable length of time?

Leaving the room as it was found

Did the learner:

- Return all furniture, food and animals to the room after spraying?
- Remove all covers fixed before spraying?

| | Yes | No | Remarks |

Collection of mosquitos

Did the learner:

- Collect the mosquitos in a systematic way from the spray sheets, starting from the doorway?
- Collect all the mosquitos from the spray sheets?
- Assemble the mosquito containers correctly, with cotton wool and filter paper?
- Pick up all specimens with forceps and transfer them to containers, without loss or damage?
- Pack specimens correctly, to prevent them from drying out?

Record-keeping

Did the learner record legibly and with complete accuracy:

- location of the house?
- date and time of collection?
- house number and/or householder's name?
- type of building?
- number of people or animals in the room during the previous night?
- whether the house had been sprayed previously, and, if so, the date of the last spraying?
- his or her own name?
- times when collecting started and finished?
- the number of mosquitos collected?

Departure

- Did the learner thank the householder for his or her assistance?

Overall assessment of learner's performance and feedback report

The following aspects of the learner's performance are quite satisfactory and need no further improvement:

The following aspects of the learner's performance are in need of improvement, and my specific recommendations for achieving this are:

Name of learner   **Name of tutor**

Date

Outdoor collection of mosquitos

General learning objective

To be able to collect adult mosquitos resting outdoors in natural and artificial shelters

---

Teaching and learning methods

Give the learners clear demonstrations of the following procedures:

- collecting techniques using sucking tubes and hand nets in natural resting sites
- positioning of drop nets and collecting mosquitos from them
- setting up a barrel as an artificial shelter, either in a naturally shady position or covering its top with straw to provide shade
- digging a pit in the ground, about 1.5 m long × 1 m wide × 1.5 m deep, with a few holes excavated in the side walls as resting sites for mosquitos; the pit may be covered with thatch as shown in Fig. 14 in the Learner's Guide.

The learners should be requested to practise the above techniques in groups for set periods, and in groups and as individuals in a number of different sites.

When returning to field practice at a later date, the learners should be requested to collect mosquitos from both barrel and pit shelters. Alternatively, if the area you use for training is also used for routine observations and is already equipped with artificial outdoor shelters, the learners should collect from these on the day set for outdoor collecting.

All blood-fed mosquitos should be brought to you by the learners soon after collection so that they may be identified and then squashed on filter paper (for precipitin testing after dispatch to the laboratory).

Guidelines for assessment

This section involves refinement of the following skills:

- collecting mosquitos using a sucking tube
- labelling and transporting specimens.

These skills can be assessed using approaches suggested in previous Units. The major emphasis here should be an assessment of the learners' proficiency in the following new skills:

- collecting mosquitos using hand nets and drop nets
- describing the most appropriate sites for collecting and the types of artificial shelter most likely to yield large numbers of mosquitos.

The following guidelines are suggested:

- To assess the learners' choice of collecting sites, provide some brief descriptions of different vectors and ask that choices be made on the basis of the relevant Unit in the Learner's Guide.
- The new skills involved in the present Unit may be assessed using the performance appraisal form (see below).

Performance appraisal form for collecting mosquitos outdoors and from artificial shelters

You should carefully observe what each learner does and complete the form reproduced below. Your observations should be discussed with the learner and used as a basis for improving his or her performance.

	Yes	No	Remarks

Collecting outdoors using a sucking tube

Did the learner:

- Assemble the sucking tube correctly?
- Hold the sucking tube correctly?
- Suck gently and quickly without damaging the mosquitos?
- Transfer the mosquitos to paper cups without loss or damage?

Collecting outdoors using a hand net

Did the learner:

- Use the hand net in an appropriate way?
- Collect mosquitos and transfer them to paper cups without loss or damage?

Collecting mosquitos by means of a drop net

Did the learner:

- Position the drop net appropriately?
- Collect *all* the mosquitos trapped in the net?
- Transfer them all to a paper cup without loss or damage?

Collecting mosquitos from outdoor shelters

Did the learner:

- Select the most appropriate shelters for collecting?
- Select appropriate outdoor sites even if they were difficult to approach and inspect?
- Observe all normal personal precautions regarding snakes and other wild animals?
- Collect *all* mosquitos from the outdoor shelters without loss?
- Transfer *all* mosquitos to paper cups without loss or damage?

Labelling and recording

Did the learner:

- Record with complete accuracy the number of collections made outdoors?

33

	Yes	No	Remarks

- Record with complete accuracy the number of shelters examined outdoors?
- Always record to the nearest minute the time spent searching for mosquitos outdoors?
- Record the number of mosquitos in each separate drop net catch?
- Always record his or her name, the date, the time of collection, the location, the name of the nearest village, and whether insecticides had been used?

Overall assessment of learner's performance and feedback report

The following aspects of the learner's performance are quite satisfactory and need no further improvement:

The following aspects of the learner's performance are in need of further improvement, and my specific recommendations for achieving this are:

Name of learner   **Name of tutor**

Date

Direct catches of mosquitos from bait

General learning objective

To be able to make night-time collections of biting mosquitos by direct catches from human and animal baits

The collection of biting mosquitos from human and animal baits both indoors and outdoors, and the preparation of specimens for transportation to the laboratory for processing, are important aspects of entomological field work.

The collecting technique is similar whether the bait is human or animal. It consists of siting the bait in a suitable location and collecting the mosquitos with a sucking tube. In the case of human bait, however, it is desirable to capture mosquitos before they have actually bitten, so as to avoid infection with malaria parasites or other pathogens. This precaution is not necessary for animal baits.

Two methods of direct collecting from human bait are described: the individual doing the collecting or a local inhabitant may serve as the bait. The amount of malaria in an area depends partly on the number of vector mosquitos that bite humans. The collection of specimens biting humans is a method of assessing human/vector contact.

Teaching and learning methods

It is suggested that you divide the learners into three groups: one catching mosquitos from human bait indoors; another collecting from human bait sited outdoors; and a third collecting mosquitos directly from animals and from vegetation in their vicinity. Learners should spend at least two hours on each of these activities; you may wish to give appropriate demonstrations before these sessions. After the practical exercises in collecting mosquitos and preparing them for transportation, it is useful to bring all the learners together, in the field or in the classroom, whichever is more convenient, and to discuss any difficulties they have experienced. Your responses to their comments should help the learners to become more effective night-time collectors.

Guidelines for assessment

Inspection of the learning objectives for this Unit of the training programme shows that the only new skills concern the preparation of human and animal bait. All the other skills (catching mosquitos, and labelling, preparing and transporting specimens) should have been thoroughly mastered by this stage. You may use the previous guidelines for assessment of these well-established skills, although it may no longer be necessary to assess learners every time they go into the field. The following guideline is suggested for assessing the new skills:

- You could develop a simple performance appraisal form along the lines indicated earlier. This could be used to assess learners' skills in using themselves or other people as bait and in using animals for the same purpose. Attention should be paid to the safety of both the humans and the animals involved.

Collecting mosquitos in baited trap nets

General learning objective

To undertake night-time collecting of mosquitos by means of trap nets containing human or animal baits

The methods of setting up the traps and collecting mosquitos are detailed in the Learner's Guide, and are the same as for the direct collection of biting mosquitos.

With human-baited trap nets it is important to realize that mosquitos leave the outer net if they are unable to feed on bait protected by an inner bed net. It is therefore desirable that collections be made regularly during the night. The Learner's Guide specifies intervals between successive collections which vary according to season, i.e. according to whether the mosquito population density is high, moderate or low. However, even when collections are to be made hourly, those people acting as bait will have the opportunity to sleep if just one person is made responsible for collecting from several trap nets.

Teaching and learning methods

Demonstrate to the learners how baited trap nets are set up. Divide the learners into two or three groups, and ask them to start collecting at dusk. It is important that you observe carefully what each group and each individual learner does. Correct any errors that you see being made in collecting, labelling and record-keeping, and in the preparation of specimens for transportation to the laboratory.

Guidelines for assessment

There are no new skills to be acquired in this Learning Unit: the learning objectives clearly indicate that all the required skills should have been mastered in previous parts of the training programme. Since the learners are approaching the end of their training, it is important for you to concentrate mainly on any who lack proficiency in basic skills, namely: collecting mosquitos quickly without damaging them; transferring them to containers without loss or damage; accurately and completely recording all specimens collected, using appropriate forms; and preparing specimens for transportation and getting them to the laboratory in excellent condition. The following guideline is suggested for assessment of these basic skills:

- Identify learners who are weak in one or more of these skills. Develop and use a performance appraisal form covering all important aspects of the skills on the basis indicated in earlier Units.

Collecting mosquitos from exit traps

> ## General learning objective
>
> To be able to use exit traps to collect mosquitos leaving houses or animal shelters

Teaching and learning methods

Ask the learners to obtain the permission of a householder to install exit traps. They must be able to explain clearly and simply why they are collecting mosquitos, and why the occupants of the house should leave the windows containing the traps open throughout the period of collection.

It is important that the learners place and fix the exit traps correctly. You could initially demonstrate how to fix an exit trap and block other large openings in the room. A learner should then be asked to give a demonstration to the group, during which you should assess and comment on his or her performance. Divide the learners into two or three small groups and ask each to fix exit traps in different houses. Inspect their work and provide critical feedback.

Emphasis should be placed on the correct fixing of the traps because this is the only new skill involved in this Unit of the training programme. All the other required skills should have been mastered previously.

Guidelines for assessment

Assessment and evaluation should focus on remedial instruction for any learners who lack proficiency in the basic skills of collecting, transfer, recording of specimens, and transportation. In addition, you should carefully assess each learner's skill in fixing exit traps because badly fitted traps will compromise the quality of mosquito collecting. The following guidelines for assessment are suggested:

- Identify learners who lack proficiency in any of the basic skills noted above; develop and use a performance appraisal form covering these skills, as suggested earlier.
- Develop a special performance appraisal form for assessing each learner's ability to block large openings into a room, prepare the room for collecting, and fix exit traps correctly.

Notes

Collecting larvae and pupae from breeding sites

General learning objective

To be able to collect mosquito larvae and pupae from breeding sites

In larval survey work it is essential to have an adequate sketch map of the area being covered. The map should show major topographical features so that the location and extent of water sources can be marked. It is suggested that very simple sketch maps of the study area be given to the learners.

Although there are many reasons for conducting a larval survey, the field exercise should be confined to:

- confirming the species present
- determining their preferred breeding sites.

The assistance of laboratory staff should be arranged to identify the specimens collected by the learners.

The different collecting methods are described in detail in the Learner's Guide. When training has been completed, the learners should know where and how to look for anopheline larvae. Once the breeding site to be examined has been identified, the learners should know which part of the water to examine (e.g. edges of streams with slow-moving water, shady banks, hoof-prints).

The right type and size of collecting equipment should be used, depending on the nature of the breeding place, and a sufficient number of dips should be made. Each type of breeding place should be carefully recorded and larvae from each should be placed in separate bottles and accurately labelled.

Teaching and learning methods

This section of the training programme is important because it introduces learners to a range of new skills relating to the collection, recording, killing, preservation and transportation of mosquito larvae and pupae.

It is suggested that for each part of this Unit you should:

- Give a demonstration to the learners.
- Ask one or two of the more confident learners to give a demonstration to the class. You or the observing learners may comment on the quality of the demonstrator's performance and suggest improvements, bearing in mind that it is good practice to focus attention first on things done well by the

learner and then to comment on some of the things that could have been done better.

- Provide plenty of opportunities for each learner to practise all the skills involved in this part of the training. It may be helpful to divide the learners into pairs. One learner in each pair should give a demonstration while the other observes and gives feedback; the roles can then be reversed. The advantage of this practical approach is that it encourages the learners to be supportive and helpful to each other.

Guidelines for assessment

As noted above, a substantial range of new skills is introduced in this Unit. If the learners are to become proficient in collecting, recording, killing, preserving and transporting specimens, they must be adequately assessed in each of these activities. The following guidelines for assessment are suggested:

- Develop and use a performance appraisal form for all the required skills, and use it as a means of assessing each learner. An example of such a form follows these guidelines.
- Inspect all samples of larvae and pupae arriving at the laboratory. On the basis of these inspections, provide feedback to the learners about the appropriateness of their methods of preparing and transporting specimens for identification.

Performance appraisal form for collecting, recording, killing, preserving and transporting mosquito larvae and pupae

You should carefully observe what each learner does and complete the form reproduced below. Your observations should be discussed with the learner as a means of improving his or her performance.

	Yes	No	Remarks

Searching for anopheline larvae

Did the learner:

- Choose the most likely breeding sites to look for larvae?

- Examine *all* these sites systematically and carefully?

Collecting anopheline larvae

Did the learner:

- Choose the correct instruments for collecting at the different types of breeding site?

- Use a dipper carefully and gently so as to avoid disturbing the breeding site?

- Use a dipper in the approved manner?

- Use a larval net in the approved manner?

- Use a well net in the approved manner?

Maintaining accurate records of collections

Did the learner:

- Draw an accurate sketch map of the area where the specimens were collected and assign a number to the area?

- Record the location, type of breeding place, number of dips made, date, and her or his name?

- Ensure that the number on the container holding the larvae corresponded to the number in her or his notebook?

- Ensure that all data were recorded in pencil and not with a ballpoint pen?

Assessment of record-keeping

- Were all records maintained accurately?

Killing and preserving larvae and pupae and transporting live and dead specimens

Did the learner:

- Kill larvae and pupae correctly?

	Yes	No	Remarks

- Preserve larvae and pupae in appropriate containers containing 70% alcohol?
- Label specimen containers accurately and completely?
- Ensure that live specimens had enough air to breathe?
- Ensure a supply of fresh air to containers as necessary during transportation?
- Transport larvae and pupae in a manner that restricted their movement?
- Obtain feedback on the number of live specimens sent to the laboratory and on the percentage arriving alive and in good condition?

Overall assessment of learner's performance and feedback report

The following aspects of the learner's performance are quite satisfactory and need no further improvement:

The following aspects of the learner's performance require further improvement, and my specific recommendations for achieving this are:

Name of learner   **Name of tutor**

Date

Commonly used teaching methods and their purposes

Teaching method	Purposes
Audio tapes May be used with large or small groups of learners or by the individual learner.	• To guide practical work. • As a variation in the method of presentation of material. • For the acquisition of new knowledge.
"Brainstorming" Intensive discussion focusing on a single problem. Participants are asked to develop as many solutions as possible to a problem within a limited time — generally not more than 10 minutes. No critical evaluation of solutions is offered.	• For developing new and creative ideas. • As a prelude to detailed, in-depth problem-solving.
"Buzz-groups" Groups of 2–4 people discuss a particular topic for a short time — generally no more than 5 minutes — within the context of a large-group lecture.	• To encourage all learners to participate. • To develop group cohesion and encourage learners to help one another. • To "rehearse" understanding and thus consolidate factual learning. • To stimulate creative thinking.
Case discussion Real or hypothetical problems are analysed in detail. Learners are encouraged to find solutions and make decisions.	• To help in understanding the facts underlying the problems and to eliminate misconceptions. • To show how various principles are applied to real problems.
Controlled discussion Under the control of the tutor, learners are encouraged to ask questions, raise problems and make comments following a lecture.	• To provide further consolidation of factual learning. • To bring together and synthesize the contents of a lecture and provide feedback to tutor and learners.

Teaching method	Purposes
Demonstrations Certain procedures are performed by the tutor to demonstrate skills that must be acquired by learners.	• To help develop learners' power of observation. • To provide knowledge of principles as a prelude to learners practising the skills for themselves.
Video tapes	• For development of skills in interviewing, counselling, etc. • To allow learners to see themselves "in action". • To provide learners with direct feedback.
Free group discussion Discussion in which the content and direction are principally under the learners' control. The role of the tutor is that of an observer.	• To develop effective small-group functioning. • To help learners establish the practice of self-learning. • To allow the tutor to observe developments in the learners' problem-solving skills.
Group tutorial Tutorial with 12–15 learners. The subject and direction are usually, but not invariably, under the control of the tutor.	• To facilitate understanding of particular topics, and bring together ideas. • To develop group-functioning skills.
Projects Varied in format and content, but generally submitted as a written exercise by a small group of learners or by individuals.	• To develop skills in gathering, organizing, applying and illustrating information in the context of a particular problem. • To provide practice in the presentation of data.
Private reading	• To assist in acquiring and understanding new information. • To assist the development of critical thinking skills. • To develop an ability to select and retrieve relevant information.

Teaching method	Purposes
Role-playing Learners are assigned or select certain roles (e.g. village leader, mosquito collector), then create and act out typical situations. It is essential that the content of the role-play is discussed at length by participants and observers; without this, the exercise has little value.	• To develop "self-awareness", i.e. to help the learner appreciate the effect that his or her attitudes have on other people. • To improve attitudes and behaviour by encouraging the learner to "get into the skin" of another person.
Seminar Presentation of material by one learner to a group of fellow learners, followed by critical analysis and discussion. It is not essential that the tutor be present.	• To present new information. • To help with understanding of new material.
Individual tasks The type of task assigned to the individual learner may vary, but it will generally be a problem to be solved within or outside the classroom situation.	• To foster active, direct learning. • To develop problem-solving skills. • To provide a context in which the tutor can help learners to remedy particular weaknesses.
Lecture The "classical" lecture is an uninterrupted talk by the tutor to a group of learners, generally lasting about 1 hour. The form may be modified and used in conjunction with "buzz groups", syndicate groups, etc.	• To transmit information. • To impart general background knowledge of a particular subject. • To synthesize a wide variety of information into a coherent whole.
Practical classes Learners perform experiments, write up their results, and draw appropriate conclusions.	• To develop powers of observation. • To develop familiarity with equipment and skill in its use. • To develop problem-solving through collection, analysis and evaluation of data.
Problem-centred groups Problem-solving in the classroom situation by groups of 4–8 learners, partly under the direction of the tutor.	• To develop skills in analysing and solving problems and in decision-making. • For practice in applying theoretical knowledge to "real" problems.

Teaching method	Purposes
Step-by-step lecture A lecture format linked to and organized around, for example, a set of 35-mm slides or a number of multiple-choice questions.	• To impart new information and reinforce its understanding.
Step-by-step discussion Working with a small group (8–10) of learners, the tutor directs a discussion centred on a particular issue or a set of pre-prepared questions. The intention is to draw out from the learners the required information.	• To present new factual material. • To help learners in the process of scientific and deductive reasoning and of drawing appropriate conclusions.
Syndicate group The class is divided into groups of 4–6 people; all groups work on the same, or closely related, problems, with occasional teacher contact. Each group prepares a report, which is presented to the rest of the class. The syndicate group technique can be used in conjunction with tutorials.	• To develop skills in seeking out, organizing and presenting information. • To foster cooperation between learners in planning, writing and presenting a report.

Questionnaire for evaluation of training

Instructions for completion of questionnaire

Use the following code to indicate the extent to which you agree or disagree with each of the statements made in the questionnaire:

1 Disagree strongly
2 Disagree
4 Agree
5 Agree strongly.

These numbers are printed alongside each question. You should circle the number that corresponds most closely to your opinion.

The difference between options 1 and 2 and between options 4 and 5 is one of degree only. To oblige you to express a definite opinion, no code 3 has been included (except for question 12); this allows a "satisfaction index" to be calculated for each question.

Take your time over completing the questionnaire. You do not have to put your name on it if you would rather not, but *please answer the questions as frankly as possible.*

Section I. Overall assessment of the training activity

1. Overall, the organization of the training programme was satisfactory.

   1 2 4 5

2. The training programme covered all the subject matter in adequate detail. (If you disagree with this, state which subjects should have been given greater coverage.)

   1 2 4 5

   Comments:

   _____
   _____
   _____
   _____
   _____
   _____

3. The tutors and facilitators for this training course had sufficient knowledge and teaching ability to provide you with the necessary skills and competence.

   1 2 4 5

Comments:

_____

_____

_____

_____

_____

_____

4. The time allocated to each part of the training was adequate relative to the total time available. (If you disagree with this, state which particular topic should have been allotted more or less time.)   1 2 4 5

Comments:

_____

_____

_____

_____

_____

_____

Section II. Relevance and usefulness of the different teaching methods

5. Overall, the teaching methods used in this training course were effective.   1 2 4 5

6. The use of the various teaching methods listed below was quite appropriate.

Large group presentations   1 2 4 5

Comments:

_____

_____

_____

_____

_____

Practical demonstrations (laboratory)   1 2 4 5

Comments:

_____

_____

_____

_____

_____

Laboratory work and facilities (including equipment)   1 2 4 5

Comments:

_____
_____
_____
_____
_____
_____

Field work   1 2 4 5

Comments:

_____
_____
_____
_____
_____
_____

Small group discussions   1 2 4 5

Comments:

_____
_____
_____
_____
_____
_____

Self-study   1 2 4 5

Comments:

_____
_____
_____
_____
_____
_____

Quizzes, tests and other evaluation exercises   1 2 4 5

Comments:

_____
_____
_____
_____
_____
_____

Section III. Assessment of teaching materials

7. The audiovisual materials (slides, overhead projection transparencies) used in the training were very helpful.   1   2   4   5

    Suggestions for improvement:

    _____
    _____
    _____
    _____
    _____
    _____

8. The teaching materials provided were satisfactory in all respects.   1   2   4   5

    Suggestions for improvement:

    _____
    _____
    _____
    _____
    _____
    _____

Section IV. Implementation of training; attitude of tutor and facilitators

9. The general atmosphere of the training course made this a good learning experience.   1   2   4   5

    Comments:

    _____
    _____
    _____
    _____
    _____
    _____

10. Every effort was made to help you achieve the learning objectives.   1   2   4   5

    Comments:

    _____
    _____
    _____
    _____
    _____
    _____

11. You were able to achieve all the learning objectives of the training programme.

1 2 4 5

Comments:

_____
_____
_____
_____
_____
_____

Section V. Overall evaluation of the training

12. What overall rating would you give to this training programme? (Circle your response.)

  1   2   3   4   5
Lowest   Highest

13. With regard to this training experience, state the following (giving actual examples):

(a) the three aspects that impressed you *most favourably*

_____
_____
_____
_____
_____
_____

(b) the three aspects that impressed you *least favourably*

_____
_____
_____
_____
_____
_____

14. Do you have any additional comments regarding any aspect of the training programme? If so, please make them below.

_____
_____
_____
_____
_____

Analysing responses to the questionnaire

The following method will allow you to analyse the responses to the questionnaire quite simply and quickly. Take a fresh (uncompleted) copy of the questionnaire; against each question, mark the learners' responses. For example:

5. Overall, the teaching methods used in this training course were effective.

This shows that two learners considered the teaching methods were not effective while 28 agreed that they were effective.

Now multiply the number of answers by the corresponding coefficient:

$$(2 \times 2) + (10 \times 4) + (18 \times 5) = 4 + 40 + 90 = \mathbf{134}$$

The "satisfaction index" is calculated as a percentage. For the above example, the number 134 is multiplied by 20 (i.e. 100 divided by the maximum coefficient, 5) and divided by 30 (the number of learners):

$$\frac{134 \times 20}{30} = 89.3\%$$

Since the satisfaction index is calculated in such a way that 60% represents "average" satisfaction, you should make a note of any questions for which the index is below 60%. (If there is none, identify the five questions for which the index is lowest and the five for which it is highest.) Let the learners know the results of this questionnaire at the final evaluation session on the last day of the training programme.